While every precaution has been taken in the preparation of this book, the publisher assumes no responsibility for errors or omissions, or for damages resulting from the use of the information contained herein.

TRIMMING TRIUMPH

First edition. February 2, 2024.

Copyright © 2024 Marko Nikolic.

ISBN: 979-8224219049

Written by Marko Nikolic.

TRIMMING TRIUMPH: A HOLISTIC GUIDE TO SUSTAINABLE WEIGHT LOSS

MENTAL CLARITY THROUGH PRODUCTIVE HABITS

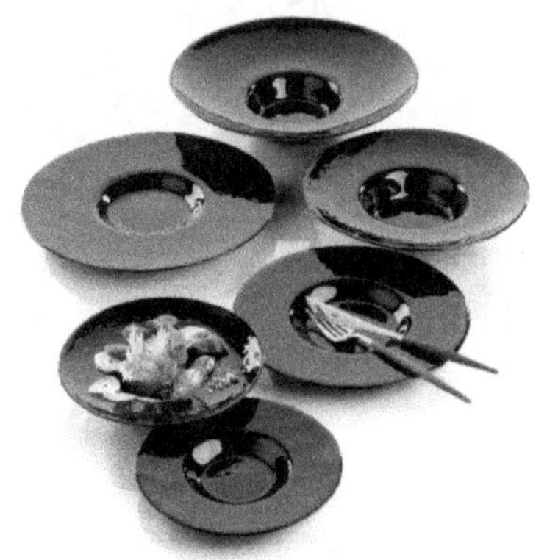

IMPROVE YOUR HEALTH TODAY!

INTRODUCTION

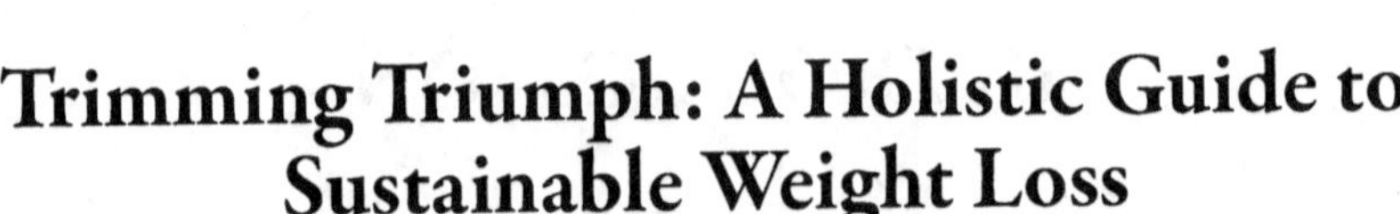

Trimming Triumph: A Holistic Guide to Sustainable Weight Loss

Welcome to "Trimming Triumph," your comprehensive guide to achieving lasting success in your weight loss journey. In this ebook, we will embark on a transformative exploration of holistic approaches to wellness, combining effective strategies for physical, mental, and emotional well-being. Get ready to discover the keys to sustainable weight loss that goes beyond quick fixes, fad diets, and restrictive measures.

Chapter 1: Setting the Foundation

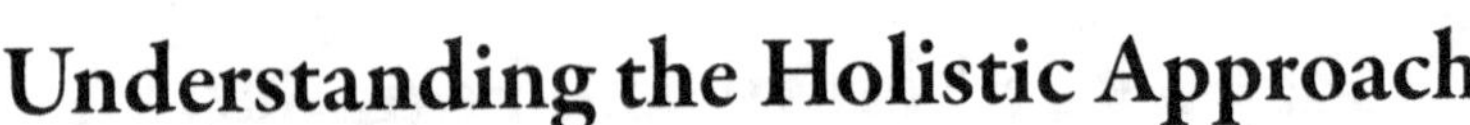

Understanding the Holistic Approach

In the realm of weight loss, the term "holistic approach" has become increasingly prominent, emphasizing a comprehensive understanding of the interconnected aspects of an individual's well-being. Far beyond merely focusing on the number on the scale, the holistic approach considers the mind, body, and spirit as integral components in the journey towards sustainable weight loss.

1. Holistic Wellness Defined:

At its core, holistic wellness involves the recognition that health is not solely determined by physical factors but is an intricate interplay of various dimensions. This approach recognizes the mind-body connection, understanding that mental and emotional well-being significantly impacts one's physical health. In the context of weight loss, this means acknowledging that factors such as stress, emotional eating, and mindset play pivotal roles in achieving lasting results.

2. Embracing the Mind-Body Connection:

The holistic approach encourages individuals to view themselves as complete beings, understanding that mental and emotional states can influence physical health. Stress, for instance, triggers the release of cortisol, a hormone that can contribute to weight gain. Through practices like mindfulness and stress management, individuals can address these factors, creating a more conducive environment for successful weight loss.

3. Personalized Strategies for Individual Needs:

Holistic weight loss recognizes that there is no one-size-fits-all solution. Each person is unique, with distinct physical, emotional, and lifestyle considerations. This approach involves tailoring strategies to fit individual needs, preferences, and circumstances. Whether it's finding enjoyable forms of exercise, crafting a personalized nutrition plan, or addressing emotional triggers, the holistic approach empowers individuals to create a weight loss strategy that resonates with their specific journey.

4. Beyond Quick Fixes:

One of the distinguishing features of the holistic approach is its departure from quick fixes and temporary solutions. Instead, it encourages sustainable lifestyle changes that contribute to long-term well-being. Crash diets and extreme workouts may yield rapid results, but the holistic perspective emphasizes building habits that are not only effective in the short term but are also maintainable over the course of a lifetime.

5. The Role of Holistic Professionals:

Holistic wellness often involves collaboration with professionals from various fields. Nutritionists, fitness trainers, mental health experts, and other holistic practitioners work together to address all facets of an individual's health. This collaborative effort ensures a more comprehensive and well-rounded approach to weight loss, considering not only the physical aspects but also the emotional and mental components.

Conclusion:

In essence, understanding the holistic approach to weight loss involves recognizing the intricate dance between mind, body, and spirit. By embracing the interconnectedness of these elements, individuals embark on a journey that goes beyond shedding pounds; it becomes a transformative process that fosters overall well-being. The holistic approach empowers individuals to not only achieve their weight loss goals but also to cultivate a sustainable and fulfilling lifestyle. As we delve deeper into the holistic principles, the subsequent chapters will explore how to apply these concepts practically, creating a roadmap for a successful and holistic weight loss journey.

Establishing Realistic Goals

In the pursuit of weight loss, establishing realistic goals serves as a cornerstone for success. A well-crafted set of objectives not only provides direction but also fosters motivation and a sense of accomplishment along the journey. This chapter delves into the importance of setting realistic goals, understanding the components of effective goal-setting, and how to navigate the path towards achieving these milestones.

1. The Significance of Realistic Goals:

Setting realistic goals is more than a mere formality; it is a fundamental aspect of a successful weight loss journey. Realistic goals are those that align with your individual capabilities, resources, and lifestyle. They take into account your starting point, acknowledging both your strengths and potential challenges. Unlike overly ambitious or vague objectives, realistic goals are attainable, creating a sense of accomplishment that propels you forward.

2. SMART Goals:

A widely recognized framework for effective goal-setting is the SMART criteria: Specific, Measurable, Achievable, Relevant, and Time-bound. Specific goals provide clarity on what you want to achieve, measurable goals allow for tracking progress, achievable goals ensure they are realistic, relevant goals align with your broader objectives, and time-bound goals set a timeframe for achievement. Applying the SMART framework ensures that your goals are well-defined and conducive to successful weight loss.

3. Short-term vs. Long-term Goals:

Breaking down your weight loss journey into short-term and long-term goals is essential for maintaining focus and motivation. Short-term goals serve as stepping stones, providing a roadmap for the immediate future. These can be weekly or monthly targets, such as increasing daily steps or trying a new healthy recipe. Long-term goals, on the other hand, encompass the broader vision of your weight loss journey. These might include achieving a specific weight, completing a fitness challenge, or cultivating a sustainable healthy lifestyle.

4. Embracing Progress, Not Perfection:

It's crucial to embrace the concept that progress, no matter how small, is a step in the right direction. Perfection is an unrealistic standard that often leads to frustration and demotivation. Celebrate the incremental victories, whether it's losing a few pounds, consistently following a workout routine, or making healthier food choices. This positive reinforcement reinforces the belief that your efforts are making a difference and fuels your commitment to the journey ahead.

5. Adjusting Goals Along the Way:

Flexibility in goal-setting is key to adapting to the dynamic nature of the weight loss process. As you progress, factors such as changes in lifestyle, unexpected challenges, or evolving fitness levels may necessitate adjustments to your goals. Being open to reassessing and modifying your objectives ensures that they remain relevant and achievable, preventing discouragement in the face of unforeseen circumstances.

6. Building a Holistic Vision:

While weight-related goals are central, it's important to adopt a holistic perspective. Consider incorporating goals related to mental and emotional well-being, such as stress management, improved sleep, and enhanced self-care. A comprehensive vision addresses the interconnected aspects of health, fostering a more balanced and sustainable approach to weight loss.

Conclusion:

Establishing realistic goals is the bedrock of a successful weight loss journey. By embracing the principles of specificity, measurability, achievability, relevance, and time-bound criteria, individuals can create a roadmap that guides them towards both short-term milestones and long-term transformation. As we move forward, the subsequent chapters will explore practical strategies for setting and achieving realistic goals, ensuring that your journey towards sustainable weight loss is not only effective but also fulfilling and empowering.

Embracing a Positive Mindset

In the intricate tapestry of weight loss, the thread of mindset weaves a powerful narrative. Embracing a positive mindset is not merely a motivational cliché; it is a foundational element that can significantly influence the trajectory of your journey towards sustainable weight loss. This chapter explores the profound impact of mindset, strategies to cultivate a positive mental outlook, and the role it plays in navigating challenges along the way.

1. The Mind-Body Connection:

The intricate interplay between the mind and body is a central theme in the pursuit of weight loss. A positive mindset can be a catalyst for physical well-being, influencing behaviors, habits, and even physiological responses. Conversely, a negative mindset can create barriers, contributing to stress, emotional eating, and self-sabotage. Recognizing and harnessing the power of the mind-body connection is a key aspect of cultivating a positive mindset.

2. Shifting from a Fixed to a Growth Mindset:

Psychologist Carol Dweck introduced the concept of mindset, distinguishing between a fixed mindset and a growth mindset. A fixed mindset sees abilities as innate and unchangeable, while a growth mindset embraces the belief that abilities can be developed through dedication and effort. Applying a growth mindset to your weight loss journey allows for a more adaptive approach, viewing challenges as opportunities for learning and improvement rather than insurmountable obstacles.

3. Cultivating Self-Compassion:

In the pursuit of weight loss, individuals often grapple with self-criticism and unrealistic expectations. Cultivating self-compassion involves treating oneself with kindness, recognizing that setbacks are a natural part of any transformative journey. Embracing self-compassion allows for resilience in the face of challenges, fostering a positive mindset that is essential for long-term success.

4. Positive Affirmations and Visualization:

The power of positive affirmations and visualization cannot be understated. Affirmations are positive statements that reinforce desired outcomes, while visualization involves mentally picturing oneself achieving goals. Incorporating these practices into your daily routine can reshape thought patterns, instilling confidence, and reinforcing the belief that success is not only possible but inevitable.

5. Surrounding Yourself with Positivity:

The influence of external factors on mindset is profound. Surrounding yourself with a positive support system, whether it's friends, family, or like-minded individuals on a similar journey, creates an environment conducive to maintaining a positive mindset. Engaging in uplifting activities, consuming inspirational content, and seeking encouragement from others contribute to a mindset that thrives on optimism and possibility.

6. Mindful Eating and Emotional Awareness:

A positive mindset extends to the way you approach food and eating habits. Mindful eating involves being present and intentional during meals, savoring each bite, and paying attention to hunger and fullness cues. Emotional awareness, on the other hand, involves recognizing and addressing the emotional triggers that may lead to unhealthy eating patterns. By fostering a positive relationship with food, individuals can navigate their weight loss journey with a balanced and empowered mindset.

Conclusion:

Embracing a positive mindset is not a one-time endeavor; it is an ongoing practice that shapes the very foundation of your weight loss journey. As we delve into the subsequent chapters, practical strategies and techniques will be explored, empowering you to nurture a positive mindset that not only propels you towards your weight loss goals but also enriches your overall well-being. The journey towards sustainable weight loss is not just a physical transformation; it is a profound shift in mindset that opens the door to lasting change and self-discovery.

Chapter 2: Nourishing Your Body

Crafting a Balanced and Nutrient-Rich Diet

Abalanced and nutrient-rich diet forms the cornerstone of a successful and sustainable weight loss journey. This chapter explores the essential components of a well-rounded eating plan, the importance of balance, and practical strategies for incorporating nutrient-rich foods into your daily meals.

1. The Importance of Balance:

A balanced diet is a key factor in achieving and maintaining a healthy weight. It involves consuming a variety of foods from different food groups in the right proportions. The concept of balance extends beyond mere calorie counting; it encompasses the distribution of macronutrients (carbohydrates, proteins, and fats) and micronutrients (vitamins and minerals) that are vital for overall health. Striking a balance ensures that your body receives the necessary nutrients for optimal functioning while managing caloric intake.

2. Building Blocks of a Balanced Diet:

- Fruits and Vegetables: These nutrient powerhouses provide essential vitamins, minerals, fiber, and antioxidants. Aim to include a colorful array of fruits and vegetables in your meals, as different colors often indicate diverse nutritional profiles.

- Whole Grains: Incorporating whole grains such as quinoa, brown rice, and oats provides complex carbohydrates, fiber, and a range of nutrients that contribute to sustained energy levels and overall well-being.

- Lean Proteins: Protein is crucial for muscle maintenance, repair, and satiety. Include sources of lean protein, such as poultry, fish, tofu, legumes, and low-fat dairy, in your diet.

- Healthy Fats: Opt for sources of healthy fats, such as avocados, nuts, seeds, and olive oil. These fats support nutrient absorption, brain health, and provide a feeling of satiety.

- Dairy or Dairy Alternatives: Calcium-rich foods are essential for bone health. Choose dairy or fortified dairy alternatives to meet your calcium needs.

3. Portion Control and Mindful Eating:

While the quality of food is crucial, so is the quantity. Portion control plays a pivotal role in managing caloric intake. Practicing mindful eating involves paying attention to hunger and fullness cues, savoring each bite, and avoiding distractions during meals. By being more attuned to your body's signals, you can prevent overeating and foster a healthier relationship with food.

4. Hydration:

Water is often overlooked but is a fundamental component of a balanced diet. Staying adequately hydrated supports overall bodily functions, aids digestion, and can contribute to a feeling of fullness. Aim to consume an adequate amount of water throughout the day, and consider incorporating herbal teas and infused water for variety.

5. MEAL PLANNING AND Preparation:

Successful adherence to a balanced diet often involves planning and preparation. Set aside time to plan your meals, ensuring they include a variety of nutrients. Consider batch cooking or preparing ingredients in advance to streamline the cooking process, making it easier to make nutritious choices even on busy days.

6. Flexibility and Enjoyment:

While structure is important, flexibility is equally crucial for long-term adherence. Allow yourself the freedom to enjoy occasional treats and indulge in your favorite foods in moderation. This approach helps prevent feelings of deprivation and fosters a sustainable relationship with food.

Conclusion:

Crafting a balanced and nutrient-rich diet is a fundamental aspect of achieving and maintaining a healthy weight. As you embark on your weight loss journey, view your dietary choices as a positive and nourishing investment in your well-being. The subsequent chapters will delve into specific dietary strategies, tips for overcoming common challenges, and guidance on tailoring your diet to your individual needs. Remember, a balanced diet is not a restrictive set of rules but a flexible and enjoyable lifestyle choice that promotes both physical and mental wellness.

The Role of Portion Control in Weight Management

In the intricate dance of weight management, portion control emerges as a pivotal player, influencing not only the quantity of calories consumed but also the overall success of a balanced and sustainable diet. This chapter explores the significance of portion control, strategies for implementation, and its profound impact on achieving and maintaining a healthy weight.

1. Understanding Portion Control:

Portion control involves being mindful of the amount of food you consume in a single sitting. It's a nuanced approach that goes beyond rigid restrictions, encouraging a balanced and realistic view of serving sizes. The goal is not to deprive oneself but to establish a healthy relationship with food by recognizing and respecting the body's signals of hunger and fullness.

2. The Caloric Equation:

At its core, weight management is fundamentally tied to the balance between caloric intake and expenditure. Consuming more calories than the body needs leads to weight gain, while a calorie deficit results in weight loss. Portion control directly influences this equation by managing the number of calories ingested, playing a critical role in achieving and maintaining a healthy weight.

3. Visual Cues and Practical Strategies:

Effective portion control often begins with understanding visual cues and employing practical strategies. Some useful tips include:

- Use Smaller Plates: Opting for smaller plates can create an optical illusion, making portions appear larger and promoting a sense of satisfaction with less food.

- Divide Your Plate: Mentally dividing your plate into sections for proteins, vegetables, and carbohydrates can guide you in creating a balanced and proportionate meal.

- Mindful Eating Practices: Paying attention to the act of eating, savoring each bite, and eating without distractions can enhance awareness of portion sizes and prevent overeating.

- Pre-Portioning Snacks: Rather than eating directly from a larger package, pre-portioning snacks into smaller containers can prevent mindless overconsumption.

4. Overcoming the Super-Size Culture:

Modern food environments often promote larger portion sizes, contributing to the normalization of overeating. From super-sized fast-food meals to larger-than-life restaurant servings, the super-size culture can lead to distorted perceptions of appropriate portions. Recognizing and resisting these influences is crucial for effective portion control.

5. Listening to Hunger and Fullness Signals:

Portion control is not solely about external cues but also about tuning into internal signals of hunger and fullness. Learning to distinguish between physical hunger and emotional cravings allows for more intentional and mindful eating. Eating slowly and paying attention to how your body feels during and after a meal can guide portion sizes based on actual nutritional needs.

6. The Role of Nutrient Density:

Portion control is not just about limiting quantity; it's also about maximizing nutrient density. Choosing nutrient-rich foods allows you to get the most nutritional value from your meals without excess calories. Focusing on whole, unprocessed foods provides essential vitamins, minerals, and fiber, promoting satiety and overall well-being.

Conclusion:

In the tapestry of weight management, portion control is a thread that weaves through the fabric of sustainable and balanced nutrition. By understanding the nuances of portion sizes, recognizing visual cues, and embracing mindful eating practices, individuals can navigate the challenges of modern food environments. The subsequent chapters will delve deeper into practical strategies for incorporating portion control into your daily life, offering insights into meal planning, dining out, and sustaining a healthy relationship with food. Remember, portion control is not a restrictive measure but a liberating skill that empowers you to make intentional choices, fostering a journey towards lasting well-being.

Smart Food Choices for Lasting Energy

In the hustle and bustle of daily life, sustaining energy levels becomes paramount for overall well-being. This chapter explores the concept of smart food choices—selecting nutrient-dense options that provide lasting energy, enhance focus, and contribute to the maintenance of a healthy weight. From understanding the impact of different macronutrients to exploring specific foods that fuel sustained vitality, this discussion aims to empower you with the knowledge to make informed dietary decisions.

1. The Role of Macronutrients:

Macronutrients—carbohydrates, proteins, and fats—are the primary components of our diet, each playing a unique role in energy metabolism.

- Carbohydrates: Often labeled as the body's preferred energy source, carbohydrates provide readily available fuel. Opt for complex carbohydrates found in whole grains, fruits, and vegetables, as they release energy gradually, sustaining you throughout the day.

- Proteins: Essential for muscle repair and maintenance, proteins contribute to a feeling of fullness and stabilize blood sugar levels. Include lean protein sources such as poultry, fish, tofu, legumes, and dairy in your meals for sustained energy.

- Fats: Healthy fats, such as those found in avocados, nuts, seeds, and olive oil, play a crucial role in satiety and support the absorption of fat-soluble vitamins. Incorporating these fats into your diet helps sustain energy levels and promotes overall well-being.

2. Complex Carbohydrates for Sustained Energy:

Choosing complex carbohydrates over simple sugars is key to maintaining lasting energy levels. Whole grains like brown rice, quinoa, oats, and whole wheat provide a steady release of glucose into the bloodstream, preventing rapid spikes and crashes in energy. Additionally, the fiber content in these foods promotes a feeling of fullness, contributing to better appetite control.

3. Protein-Packed Choices:

Proteins are not only building blocks for muscles but also play a significant role in providing lasting energy. Including sources like lean meats, poultry, fish, eggs, legumes, and dairy in your meals helps regulate blood sugar levels and staves off feelings of hunger between meals.

4. Healthy Fats for Sustained Satiation:

Incorporating healthy fats into your diet contributes to sustained energy and satiety. Avocados, nuts, seeds, and fatty fish are rich in omega-3 fatty acids, which have been linked to improved cognitive function and mood, enhancing overall well-being.

5. Nutrient-Dense Snacking:

Smart food choices extend to snacks, which can either support or sabotage your energy levels. Opt for nutrient-dense snacks such as fresh fruit, yogurt, a handful of nuts, or whole-grain crackers with hummus. These choices provide a combination of macronutrients, keeping you energized between meals without the crash associated with sugary snacks.

6. Hydration's Role in Energy:

Staying adequately hydrated is often underestimated in its impact on energy levels. Dehydration can lead to fatigue and impaired cognitive function. Water, herbal teas, and infused water with fruits and herbs are excellent choices to maintain hydration throughout the day.

7. Balanced and Regular Meals:

Spacing your meals evenly throughout the day helps regulate blood sugar levels and sustains energy. Aim for a balanced combination of carbohydrates, proteins, and fats in each meal to provide a steady supply of nutrients and prevent energy dips.

8. Tailoring Your Diet to Your Lifestyle:

Smart food choices are not one-size-fits-all. Consider your individual needs, activity levels, and preferences when crafting your dietary plan. Whether you're an athlete requiring additional fuel for workouts or someone with a sedentary lifestyle seeking sustained energy for work, tailoring your diet to your unique circumstances is essential.

Conclusion:

Making smart food choices for lasting energy is a holistic endeavor that goes beyond merely satisfying hunger. By understanding the roles of carbohydrates, proteins, and fats and incorporating nutrient-dense options into your meals and snacks, you can cultivate sustained vitality throughout the day. The subsequent chapters will delve into practical strategies for meal planning, grocery shopping, and overcoming common challenges, ensuring that your journey towards lasting energy is both enjoyable and empowering. Remember, the choices you make in the kitchen have a profound impact on your energy levels, overall health, and the success of your weight management efforts.

Chapter 3: Igniting the Flame: Exercise for Everyone

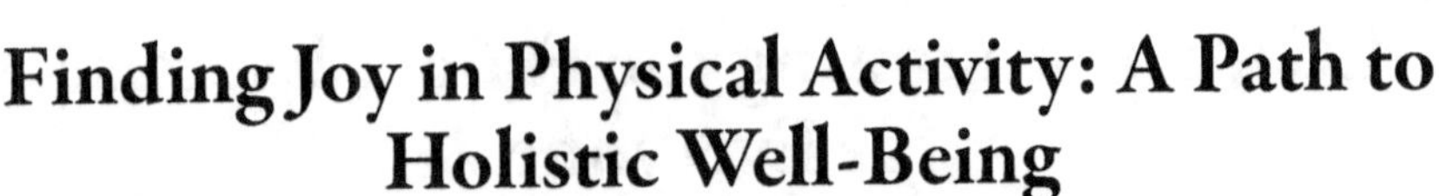

Finding Joy in Physical Activity: A Path to Holistic Well-Being

Engaging in physical activity transcends the notion of mere exercise; it's a journey towards holistic well-being that encompasses not only the physical benefits but also the joy and fulfillment that movement brings to your life. This chapter explores the importance of finding joy in physical activity, the psychological and emotional benefits, and practical strategies to make exercise an enjoyable and sustainable part of your routine.

1. The Transformative Power of Joyful Movement:

Physical activity is often framed as a means to an end—whether it be weight loss, muscle gain, or improved cardiovascular health. However, the concept of finding joy in movement shifts the focus from obligation to enthusiasm. When exercise becomes a source of joy, it transcends the realm of routine; it becomes a positive and fulfilling aspect of your lifestyle. Joyful movement fosters a positive relationship with your body, creating a mindset that is conducive to long-term engagement.

2. Unleashing the Psychological Benefits:

Beyond the physical benefits of increased strength, flexibility, and endurance, joyful movement contributes significantly to mental and emotional well-being. Regular physical activity has been linked to reduced stress, anxiety, and depression. The release of endorphins, often referred to as "feel-good" hormones, during exercise creates a natural mood boost, promoting a sense of happiness and relaxation.

3. Connecting with Intrinsic Motivation:

Finding joy in physical activity involves tapping into intrinsic motivation—doing activities because they bring personal satisfaction and pleasure rather than external rewards. This might involve exploring different forms of exercise until you find what resonates with you, whether it's dancing, hiking, yoga, or team sports. By aligning your physical activities with your personal interests and preferences, you cultivate a sustainable and enjoyable exercise routine.

4. Embracing Variety and Playfulness:

Monotony can be a significant deterrent to regular exercise. Introducing variety and playfulness into your routine not only keeps things interesting but also sparks excitement. Experiment with different forms of physical activity, join group classes, or incorporate playful elements like dance, games, or outdoor activities. By making movement enjoyable, you're more likely to stick with it over the long term.

5. Setting Realistic and Enjoyable Goals:

Setting goals for physical activity is essential, but they need not be solely performance-based or focused on external outcomes. Consider setting goals that revolve around the joy of movement, such as trying a new activity, spending more time in nature, or achieving a personal best in a favorite exercise. These goals shift the emphasis from external validation to personal satisfaction, fostering a positive relationship with physical activity.

6. Mindful Movement and Presence:

Engaging in mindful movement involves being fully present and attentive during exercise. Whether it's focusing on the sensation of your breath during yoga, appreciating the scenery during a walk, or enjoying the rhythm of your movements, mindfulness enhances the joy of physical activity. This approach not only deepens the connection between mind and body but also makes the experience more meaningful and enjoyable.

7. Social Engagement:

Physical activity can be a social endeavor, amplifying the joy through shared experiences. Whether it's joining a sports team, participating in group fitness classes, or simply taking walks with friends, the social element adds a layer of enjoyment and accountability, making exercise a social event rather than a solitary task.

8. Celebrating Progress and Milestones:

Celebrate the progress you make in your physical activity journey, no matter how small. Recognize and acknowledge the improvements in your strength, endurance, or flexibility. By celebrating milestones, you reinforce the positive association with movement, making it a joyful and fulfilling part of your life.

Conclusion:

Finding joy in physical activity is not just about breaking a sweat; it's about creating a positive and enriching experience that contributes to your overall well-being. As you embark on this journey, remember that movement should bring you joy, not stress. The subsequent chapters will delve into practical strategies for incorporating joyful movement into your daily life, overcoming obstacles, and making physical activity an integral and sustainable part of your holistic wellness routine. By infusing joy into your approach to exercise, you're not just enhancing your physical health; you're nurturing a positive and lasting relationship with movement that will contribute to a fulfilling and vibrant life.

Incorporating Exercise into Your Daily Routine

Exercise is a cornerstone of a healthy lifestyle, offering a myriad of physical, mental, and emotional benefits. This chapter explores the importance of regular physical activity, strategies for incorporating exercise into your daily routine, and the transformative impact it can have on your overall well-being.

1. The Benefits of Regular Exercise:

The benefits of regular exercise extend far beyond weight management. Engaging in physical activity positively influences cardiovascular health, strengthens muscles and bones, enhances flexibility and balance, and boosts mood through the release of endorphins—our body's natural mood lifters. Additionally, exercise plays a pivotal role in stress reduction, improving sleep quality, and supporting cognitive function.

2. Finding Your Exercise Motivation:

Understanding your personal motivations for exercise is crucial for long-term commitment. Whether your goal is weight loss, stress relief, increased energy, or improved overall health, clarifying your objectives provides a clear roadmap for designing a sustainable exercise routine. Consider what activities you enjoy, as incorporating elements of fun into your routine increases the likelihood of adherence.

3. Types of Exercise:

Variety is key when it comes to exercise. Incorporate a mix of cardiovascular exercises, strength training, flexibility work, and balance exercises into your routine to ensure a well-rounded approach to fitness.

- Cardiovascular Exercises: Activities such as walking, jogging, cycling, swimming, and dancing elevate your heart rate, improving cardiovascular health and burning calories.

- Strength Training: Building and maintaining muscle mass not only contributes to a toned physique but also enhances metabolism. Include weightlifting, bodyweight exercises, or resistance training in your regimen.

- Flexibility and Balance Exercises: Incorporating activities like yoga or Pilates improves flexibility, balance, and overall body awareness, reducing the risk of injury and promoting functional movement.

4. Setting Realistic Exercise Goals:

Establishing realistic and achievable exercise goals is paramount for success. Begin with manageable targets, gradually increasing intensity and duration as your fitness level improves. Consistency is more important than intensity, especially when integrating exercise into your daily routine.

5. Scheduling Exercise:

In the midst of busy schedules, prioritizing exercise requires intentional planning. Treat your workouts as non-negotiable appointments and schedule them into your day. Whether it's morning, lunchtime, or evening, finding a consistent time that aligns with your routine enhances adherence.

6. Making Exercise Enjoyable:

Discovering activities you genuinely enjoy transforms exercise from a chore into a rewarding and enjoyable part of your day. Whether it's dancing, hiking, playing sports, or attending fitness classes, finding activities that bring joy not only ensures consistency but also fosters a positive association with physical activity.

7. Incorporating Movement Throughout the Day:

Exercise doesn't solely happen within the confines of a gym. Incorporating movement into your daily routine, such as taking the stairs, walking or biking to work, or integrating short bursts of activity during breaks, contributes to overall physical activity levels. Small, consistent efforts throughout the day add up and make a significant impact on your health.

8. Accountability and Social Support:

Enlisting the support of friends, family, or exercise partners provides accountability and motivation. Joining fitness classes, sports leagues, or online communities creates a supportive environment, making exercise a social and enjoyable experience.

9. Adapting to Changes and Overcoming Challenges:

Life is dynamic, and your exercise routine should be adaptable. Recognize that challenges may arise, such as changes in schedule, travel, or unexpected commitments. Having contingency plans and a flexible mindset helps you navigate these challenges without derailing your fitness journey.

Conclusion:

Incorporating exercise into your daily routine is a transformative commitment to your overall well-being. By understanding the benefits of regular physical activity, identifying your motivations, and adopting a varied and enjoyable approach to exercise, you pave the way for a sustainable and fulfilling fitness journey. The subsequent chapters will delve into specific exercises, strategies for overcoming common barriers, and guidance on tailoring your routine to your individual needs. Remember, the journey to a healthier, more active lifestyle is a personal and empowering adventure that extends far beyond the confines of a gym—it's about embracing movement as an integral part of your daily life.

Tailoring Workouts to Your Fitness Level

Embarking on a fitness journey is a commendable decision, and one of the keys to long-term success lies in tailoring your workouts to your current fitness level. This chapter explores the importance of understanding and respecting your fitness baseline, the benefits of gradual progression, and practical strategies for crafting a workout routine that aligns with your individual capabilities and goals.

1. Assessing Your Fitness Level:

Before diving into a workout routine, it's essential to assess your current fitness level. This involves evaluating your cardiovascular endurance, strength, flexibility, and overall stamina. Honest self-reflection and, if possible, consultations with fitness professionals can provide valuable insights into where you stand on the fitness spectrum.

2. The Importance of Gradual Progression:

One of the common pitfalls in fitness is the temptation to push oneself too hard, too soon. Gradual progression is a fundamental principle that not only reduces the risk of injury but also enhances the sustainability of your fitness journey. Starting with exercises and intensities that match your current abilities allows your body to adapt and build a strong foundation for more advanced workouts in the future.

3. Building Cardiovascular Endurance:

For those beginning their fitness journey, incorporating cardiovascular exercises at a moderate intensity is a great starting point. Brisk walking, cycling, or swimming are excellent choices. As your cardiovascular endurance improves, you can gradually increase the intensity and duration of these activities or explore more challenging options like running or high-intensity interval training (HIIT).

4. Strength Training for Beginners:

Strength training is a crucial component of a well-rounded fitness routine. For beginners, bodyweight exercises such as squats, lunges, push-ups, and planks provide a solid foundation. As you progress, you can gradually introduce resistance training using weights or resistance bands. A focus on proper form is paramount to prevent injuries and ensure the effectiveness of the exercises.

5. Flexibility and Mobility Exercises:

Flexibility and mobility are often overlooked but are essential for overall fitness and injury prevention. Incorporate stretching and mobility exercises into your routine to improve flexibility and range of motion. Yoga and Pilates are excellent options for enhancing both flexibility and core strength.

6. Listen to Your Body:

Listening to your body is a critical aspect of tailoring workouts to your fitness level. Pay attention to how your body responds to different exercises, and be mindful of any discomfort or pain. It's normal to experience muscle soreness, but sharp or persistent pain may indicate an issue that needs attention.

7. INDIVIDUALIZED GOALS:

Set realistic and individualized fitness goals based on your current capabilities and aspirations. Whether your goal is to improve cardiovascular health, build strength, or enhance flexibility, having clear objectives provides direction and motivation for your fitness journey.

8. Consistency Over Intensity:

Consistency is key to any successful fitness endeavor. Rather than focusing on intense, sporadic workouts, prioritize regular, sustainable activity. Building a habit of consistent exercise not only contributes to physical improvements but also fosters a positive mindset towards fitness.

9. Professional Guidance:

If you're unsure about designing a workout routine tailored to your fitness level, seeking guidance from fitness professionals can be immensely beneficial. Personal trainers, fitness instructors, or physical therapists can provide personalized advice, ensuring that your workouts align with your goals and physical condition.

10. Progress Tracking:

Regularly tracking your progress is a motivating tool that allows you to celebrate achievements and adjust your workouts accordingly. Whether it's noting increased endurance, higher weights lifted, or improved flexibility, recognizing your advancements reinforces a positive mindset towards fitness.

Conclusion:

Tailoring workouts to your fitness level is not a sign of limitation but a strategic approach that sets the foundation for long-term success. As you navigate your fitness journey, remember that everyone starts somewhere, and gradual progression is the key to sustained improvement. The subsequent chapters will delve into specific workout routines, tips for overcoming challenges, and strategies for maintaining motivation, ensuring that your fitness journey is not only effective but also enjoyable and fulfilling. Embrace the process, honor your current capabilities, and relish the empowering journey towards a fitter, healthier you.

Chapter 4: Mindful Eating and Emotional Wellness

Cultivating Mindfulness in Your Eating Habits

In the fast-paced modern world, mindfulness in eating habits often takes a back seat, leading to a range of issues from overeating to emotional eating. This chapter delves into the profound benefits of cultivating mindfulness in your eating habits, exploring the concept of mindful eating, practical techniques, and how this practice can positively impact your overall well-being.

1. The Essence of Mindful Eating:

Mindful eating is a practice rooted in mindfulness, encouraging a heightened awareness and presence during meals. It involves paying attention to the sensory aspects of eating, including the flavors, textures, and aromas of food. More than just a set of guidelines, mindful eating is a mindset that fosters a healthy relationship with food, addressing the emotional and psychological aspects of eating as well.

2. Breaking Free from Multitasking:

In a world of constant distractions, multitasking during meals has become the norm. Whether it's eating in front of screens, working through lunch, or consuming meals in a hurried manner, the art of savoring each bite often gets lost. Mindful eating encourages a break from this cycle, urging individuals to set aside dedicated time for meals, free from distractions. By doing so, you not only enhance the enjoyment of your food but also allow your body to register and respond to feelings of fullness.

3. Understanding Hunger and Fullness Cues:

Mindful eating involves tuning in to your body's signals of hunger and fullness. Often, the rush of daily life leads to neglecting these cues, resulting in overeating or undereating. By practicing mindfulness, you can reconnect with your body's natural signals, learning to distinguish between physical hunger and emotional cravings. This heightened awareness empowers you to make choices aligned with your body's actual needs.

4. Savoring Each Bite:

The act of eating transcends mere sustenance; it is an experience to be savored. Mindful eating encourages slowing down the pace of your meals, allowing you to fully appreciate the flavors, textures, and aromas of your food. By savoring each bite, you not only derive greater satisfaction from your meals but also promote better digestion and nutrient absorption.

5. Overcoming Emotional Eating:

Emotional eating is a common challenge, often driven by stress, boredom, or other emotional triggers. Mindful eating provides a powerful antidote to this pattern by promoting awareness of emotional cues and developing alternative coping mechanisms. Instead of turning to food as an automatic response, individuals can learn to pause, acknowledge their emotions, and make intentional choices that nurture both physical and emotional well-being.

6. Creating a Mindful Environment:

The physical environment in which you eat can significantly impact your ability to practice mindful eating. Creating a peaceful and inviting space, free from distractions, sets the stage for a more mindful experience. Whether dining alone or with others, cultivating an environment that allows you to focus on the act of eating enhances the mindful eating journey.

7. Gratitude and Connection with Food:

Mindful eating invites a sense of gratitude for the food on your plate. Taking a moment to reflect on the journey of your food—from its source to your table—deepens your connection with the nourishment it provides. This practice fosters a greater appreciation for the efforts involved in food production and reinforces a mindful approach to consumption.

8. Incorporating Mindfulness Beyond Meals:

While mindful eating is centered around meals, extending mindfulness to other aspects of your relationship with food is equally valuable. This includes mindful grocery shopping, mindful meal planning, and even being mindful of your body's signals between meals. These practices collectively contribute to a holistic and sustainable approach to mindful living.

Conclusion:

Cultivating mindfulness in your eating habits is not a restrictive practice but a transformative journey toward a healthier and more enjoyable relationship with food. The subsequent chapters will explore practical techniques to incorporate mindfulness into your daily life, offering guidance on overcoming challenges and sustaining this mindful approach. Remember, the simple act of being present during meals has the power to nourish not only your body but also your mind and spirit, fostering a harmonious and balanced approach to eating.

Managing Stress and Emotional Eating

In the complex landscape of weight management, stress and emotional eating stand as formidable challenges. This chapter explores the intricate relationship between stress, emotions, and eating behaviors, offering insights into effective strategies for managing stress and breaking the cycle of emotional eating.

1. The Stress-Eating Connection:

Stress triggers a cascade of physiological responses, including the release of cortisol, commonly known as the stress hormone. Elevated cortisol levels can influence food preferences, particularly for high-fat and sugary foods, and lead to increased calorie consumption. Understanding this connection is crucial for addressing the root causes of stress-related eating patterns.

2. Identifying Emotional Eating:

Emotional eating involves using food to cope with emotions rather than to satisfy physical hunger. It often manifests as a response to stress, sadness, boredom, or other emotional triggers. Recognizing the signs of emotional eating, such as sudden cravings for specific comfort foods or mindless eating without genuine hunger, is the first step in breaking the cycle.

3. Mindfulness and Stress Reduction Techniques:

Practicing mindfulness and stress reduction techniques can be powerful tools in managing emotional eating. Techniques such as deep breathing, meditation, and yoga can help calm the mind, reduce stress hormones, and increase awareness of emotional triggers. Integrating these practices into your routine creates a foundation for more intentional and mindful eating.

4. Building a Support System:

Seeking support from friends, family, or a therapist can provide emotional outlets and alternative coping mechanisms for stress. Building a strong support system helps create a network of individuals who understand and empathize with your struggles, providing encouragement and assistance in navigating challenging times.

5. Emotional Awareness and Journaling:

Developing emotional awareness involves recognizing and understanding your emotions without immediately turning to food for comfort. Keeping a journal to track emotions, triggers, and the circumstances surrounding emotional eating episodes can illuminate patterns and offer valuable insights into the root causes of this behavior.

6. Creating Healthy Coping Mechanisms:

Replacing food with alternative, healthier coping mechanisms is a key aspect of overcoming emotional eating. Engaging in activities that bring joy, relaxation, and a sense of accomplishment—such as hobbies, exercise, or spending time in nature—can redirect focus away from food as the primary source of comfort.

7. BUILDING A MINDFUL Eating Practice:

Mindful eating involves being present and intentional during meals, paying attention to taste, texture, and satiety cues. Incorporating mindful eating practices helps cultivate a healthier relationship with food, fostering the ability to distinguish between physical hunger and emotional cravings.

8. Nutrition and Balanced Meals:

Ensuring your body receives adequate nutrients through balanced meals can positively impact mood and stress levels. Nutrient-dense foods, such as fruits, vegetables, whole grains, and lean proteins, support overall well-being and can contribute to a more stable emotional state.

9. Preparing for Challenging Situations:

Anticipating and preparing for situations that may trigger emotional eating is a proactive strategy. Having a plan in place, such as keeping healthy snacks on hand, practicing relaxation techniques, or reaching out to a supportive friend, empowers you to navigate challenging moments without turning to food as a default coping mechanism.

10. Professional Guidance:

In cases where emotional eating is deeply ingrained or significantly impacting well-being, seeking professional guidance from a therapist, counselor, or registered dietitian can provide tailored strategies and support. Professional interventions offer personalized insights into the emotional and psychological aspects of eating behaviors.

Conclusion:

Managing stress and emotional eating is a nuanced process that involves cultivating self-awareness, building healthy coping mechanisms, and developing a mindful approach to eating. By addressing the root causes of emotional eating and implementing practical strategies, individuals can break free from the cycle of using food as a primary response to stress or emotions. The subsequent chapters will delve into specific techniques, meal planning considerations, and lifestyle adjustments that support stress management and emotional well-being, ensuring a holistic and sustainable approach to weight management. Remember, the journey towards a healthier relationship with food is not only about what you eat but also about understanding why you eat.

Building a Healthy Relationship with Food

A healthy relationship with food is not just about what you eat; it encompasses your thoughts, feelings, and behaviors surrounding food. This chapter explores the importance of fostering a positive and balanced connection with the nourishment your body needs. From understanding the impact of societal influences to practicing mindful eating, building a healthy relationship with food is a transformative journey towards sustainable well-being.

1. Understanding Influences on Food Perception:

The modern world bombards individuals with diverse and often conflicting messages about food. Media, societal norms, and cultural expectations can shape perceptions of what is considered "good" or "bad" when it comes to food choices. Recognizing and understanding these influences is the first step in building a healthy relationship with food. It involves challenging societal norms, embracing body positivity, and shifting the focus from external expectations to internal well-being.

2. Embracing Intuitive Eating:

Intuitive eating is a philosophy that encourages listening to your body's natural cues for hunger and fullness. It involves attuning yourself to internal signals rather than adhering to external diets or rigid rules. Embracing intuitive eating allows for a more flexible and enjoyable approach to food, fostering a sustainable relationship that goes beyond restrictions and guilt associated with traditional dieting.

3. Mindful Eating Practices:

Mindful eating involves being fully present during meals, savoring each bite, and paying attention to hunger and fullness cues. This practice promotes a deeper connection with the sensory experience of eating and prevents mindless or emotional eating. By slowing down and appreciating the flavors and textures of your food, you can foster a positive relationship with nourishment.

4. Breaking Free from Emotional Eating:

Understanding and addressing emotional eating is crucial for building a healthy relationship with food. Emotional eating often stems from using food as a coping mechanism for stress, boredom, or other emotions. Developing alternative strategies for dealing with emotions, such as engaging in physical activity, practicing mindfulness, or seeking support from friends and family, helps break the cycle of using food as a primary emotional outlet.

5. Ditching the Diet Mentality:

Traditional dieting often involves strict rules, deprivation, and an "all or nothing" mindset. This approach can lead to a turbulent relationship with food, fostering guilt and shame associated with deviations from the prescribed plan. Ditching the diet mentality involves adopting a more holistic and flexible approach to eating. Instead of viewing food as the enemy, it becomes a source of nourishment, pleasure, and energy.

6. Celebrating Food as Nourishment:

Food is not just fuel; it is a source of pleasure, culture, and social connection. Celebrating food as nourishment involves recognizing the positive aspects of eating beyond its nutritional value. Enjoying meals with loved ones, exploring new flavors, and embracing the cultural significance of food contribute to a holistic and positive relationship with nourishment.

7. Overcoming Food Guilt:

Feelings of guilt after eating certain foods or indulging in treats are common, but they can be detrimental to building a healthy relationship with food. Overcoming food guilt involves letting go of the notion of "good" and "bad" foods and reframing your mindset to view food choices within the context of your overall eating patterns. Allowing yourself the freedom to enjoy a variety of foods without guilt is essential for long-term well-being.

8. Seeking Professional Guidance:

For individuals facing complex issues related to food, seeking the guidance of a registered dietitian, nutritionist, or mental health professional can be invaluable. These professionals can provide personalized advice, address specific concerns, and support you in building a healthy and sustainable relationship with food.

Conclusion:

Building a healthy relationship with food is a multifaceted journey that requires self-reflection, mindfulness, and a shift in mindset. By understanding external influences, practicing intuitive and mindful eating, and embracing food as a positive and nourishing aspect of life, individuals can cultivate a relationship that supports overall well-being. The subsequent chapters will explore practical strategies for implementing these principles in your daily life, ensuring that your journey towards a healthier relationship with food is both fulfilling and empowering. Remember, your relationship with food is a lifelong journey, and every positive step contributes to your holistic well-being.

Chapter 5: The Power of Sleep

Unraveling the Connection Between Sleep and Weight Loss

In the intricate tapestry of health and well-being, the relationship between sleep and weight loss emerges as a crucial thread that often goes unnoticed. This chapter explores the intricate interplay between quality sleep and effective weight management, shedding light on the physiological mechanisms, the impact of sleep duration on metabolism, and practical strategies to optimize both sleep and weight loss.

1. The Physiology of Sleep and Weight:

The connection between sleep and weight loss is deeply rooted in the intricate workings of our physiological systems. Sleep influences hormones that regulate hunger and satiety, including ghrelin and leptin. Ghrelin, often referred to as the "hunger hormone," increases appetite, while leptin, the "satiety hormone," signals fullness. Disruptions in sleep patterns can lead to imbalances in these hormones, potentially contributing to overeating and weight gain.

2. Metabolic Impact of Sleep Deprivation:

Beyond hormonal regulation, sleep plays a pivotal role in metabolic processes. Sleep deprivation has been linked to insulin resistance, a condition where cells become less responsive to insulin, leading to elevated blood sugar levels. This insulin resistance can contribute to weight gain and an increased risk of developing type 2 diabetes. Additionally, sleep-deprived individuals may experience alterations in their food preferences, showing a tendency to choose higher-calorie, carbohydrate-rich foods.

3. Sleep Duration and Weight Loss Success:

Studies consistently highlight the correlation between adequate sleep duration and successful weight loss. Individuals with insufficient sleep may find it more challenging to adhere to dietary plans and exercise routines. The fatigue and irritability associated with sleep deprivation can lead to increased cravings for sugary and high-calorie foods as a quick energy fix, derailing weight loss efforts.

4. Quality vs. Quantity:

While the duration of sleep is important, the quality of sleep also plays a crucial role. Restorative sleep involves cycling through different sleep stages, including deep sleep and REM (rapid eye movement) sleep. These stages are essential for physical and mental rejuvenation. Poor sleep quality may impact mood, energy levels, and the ability to make healthy choices throughout the day.

5. Practical Strategies for Improving Sleep:

a. Establishing a Consistent Sleep Schedule: Going to bed and waking up at the same time every day helps regulate the body's internal clock, promoting a more consistent sleep-wake cycle.

b. Creating a Restful Sleep Environment: Ensure your bedroom is conducive to sleep by minimizing light and noise, investing in a comfortable mattress and pillows, and maintaining a cool and dark environment.

c. Limiting Screen Time Before Bed: The blue light emitted by screens can interfere with the production of the sleep hormone melatonin. Aim to limit screen time at least an hour before bedtime.

d. Practicing Relaxation Techniques: Engage in activities that promote relaxation before bedtime, such as reading, gentle stretching, or practicing mindfulness meditation.

6. The Bidirectional Relationship:

It's essential to recognize that the relationship between sleep and weight is bidirectional. While inadequate sleep can contribute to weight gain, excess weight can also exacerbate sleep-related issues, such as sleep apnea and insomnia. Addressing both aspects—improving sleep and adopting healthy lifestyle choices—is integral to achieving holistic well-being.

7. The Importance of Consistency:

Consistency is key when unraveling the connection between sleep and weight loss. Establishing healthy sleep habits and incorporating them into a consistent daily routine can yield long-term benefits. Recognizing the symbiotic relationship between sleep, nutrition, and physical activity allows for a more comprehensive approach to weight management.

Conclusion:

The connection between sleep and weight loss is a multifaceted interplay that extends beyond mere hours of rest. By understanding the physiological mechanisms at play and implementing practical strategies to improve both the quality and quantity of sleep, individuals can enhance their overall well-being and contribute to the success of their weight loss endeavors. As we delve into subsequent chapters, we'll explore additional lifestyle factors that complement the sleep-weight relationship, providing a holistic roadmap for those seeking lasting improvements in both sleep and weight. Remember, the journey towards optimal health involves nurturing your body with the care it deserves, encompassing the vital aspects of sleep, nutrition, and physical activity.

Tips for Improving Sleep Quality

Quality sleep is a cornerstone of overall well-being, impacting physical health, cognitive function, and emotional resilience. This chapter explores practical tips and strategies to enhance sleep quality, fostering a restful and rejuvenating night's sleep.

1. Establishing a Consistent Sleep Schedule:

Creating a consistent sleep schedule is fundamental to regulating your body's internal clock, known as the circadian rhythm. Aim to go to bed and wake up at the same time every day, even on weekends. This practice helps synchronize your body's natural sleep-wake cycle, promoting better sleep quality over time.

2. Creating a Relaxing Bedtime Routine:

Establishing a calming bedtime routine signals to your body that it's time to wind down. Activities such as reading a book, taking a warm bath, practicing relaxation techniques, or gentle stretching can help transition your mind and body into a state of relaxation, preparing you for restful sleep.

3. Optimizing Your Sleep Environment:

Your sleep environment plays a crucial role in the quality of your rest. Consider the following tips:

- Comfortable Mattress and Pillows: Invest in a comfortable mattress and pillows that support proper spinal alignment and reduce discomfort during sleep.

- Dark and Quiet Atmosphere: Create a dark and quiet sleep environment. Consider blackout curtains, earplugs, or a white noise machine to minimize disturbances.

- Cool Room Temperature: Maintain a cool room temperature for optimal sleep. The ideal range is typically between 60-67 degrees Fahrenheit (15-20 degrees Celsius).

4. Limiting Exposure to Screens Before Bed:

The blue light emitted by screens on phones, tablets, and computers can interfere with the production of the sleep-inducing hormone melatonin. Aim to limit screen time at least an hour before bedtime. Consider using devices with a "night mode" that reduces blue light exposure.

5. Monitoring Your Diet and Hydration:

Certain dietary choices can impact sleep. Consider the following:

- Limit Caffeine and Nicotine: Both caffeine and nicotine are stimulants that can disrupt sleep. Aim to limit consumption, especially in the hours leading up to bedtime.

- Moderate Alcohol Consumption: While alcohol might initially make you feel sleepy, it can disrupt the later stages of sleep. Limit alcohol intake, particularly in the evening.

- Be Mindful of Late-Night Eating: Avoid heavy meals close to bedtime, as they can cause discomfort and indigestion. If you're hungry, opt for a light snack.

6. Incorporating Regular Physical Activity:

Regular physical activity has been linked to improved sleep quality. Aim for at least 30 minutes of moderate exercise most days of the week. However, avoid vigorous exercise close to bedtime, as it may have a stimulating effect.

7. Managing Stress and Anxiety:

Stress and anxiety can significantly impact sleep quality. Consider incorporating stress-reducing practices into your daily routine:

- Mindfulness and Meditation: Mindfulness meditation and deep-breathing exercises can help calm the mind and reduce stress.

- Journaling: Write down any concerns or thoughts before bedtime to help clear your mind and ease anxiety.

8. Seeking Natural Light Exposure:

Exposure to natural light during the day helps regulate your circadian rhythm and improves sleep quality. Spend time outdoors, especially in the morning, to enhance your body's natural wake-sleep cycle.

9. Consulting a Healthcare Professional:

If sleep difficulties persist despite implementing these tips, it may be advisable to consult a healthcare professional. Sleep disorders, such as insomnia or sleep apnea, may require specialized intervention and treatment.

Conclusion:

Quality sleep is a vital component of a healthy lifestyle, influencing various aspects of physical and mental well-being. By incorporating these practical tips into your routine, you can create an environment conducive to restful sleep and establish habits that promote improved sleep quality over time. Experiment with these strategies, personalize them to fit your lifestyle, and prioritize the importance of sleep in your overall health and wellness journey.

Creating a Restful Sleep Environment: A Blueprint for Tranquil Nights

The quality of your sleep is intricately tied to the environment in which you rest. This chapter delves into the essential elements of crafting a restful sleep environment, providing insights into optimizing your bedroom for peaceful nights and rejuvenated mornings.

1. The Importance of Sleep Environment:

Sleep is a vital component of overall well-being, influencing physical health, cognitive function, and emotional balance. The environment in which you sleep plays a significant role in the quality of your rest. By intentionally designing a sleep-friendly space, you can create conditions that promote relaxation, reduce sleep disturbances, and contribute to a more restful night.

2. Comfortable Bedding and Mattress:

The foundation of a restful sleep environment begins with your bedding and mattress. Choose comfortable and supportive pillows, along with a mattress that suits your preferences and provides adequate spinal alignment. Investing in quality bedding not only enhances physical comfort but also signals to your brain that your sleep space is a sanctuary for relaxation.

3. Calming Color Palette:

The colors in your bedroom can have a psychological impact on your ability to unwind. Opt for a calming color palette dominated by soft, muted tones such as blues, greens, and neutrals. These colors are associated with tranquility and can create a soothing atmosphere conducive to restful sleep.

4. Dim Lighting and Blackout Curtains:

Creating a sleep-conducive environment involves managing lighting. Dim the lights in the evening to signal to your body that it's time to wind down. Consider blackout curtains to block out external sources of light, especially if you live in an urban area or are exposed to streetlights. Darkness enhances the production of melatonin, a hormone that regulates sleep-wake cycles.

5. Declutter for Serenity:

A clutter-free space promotes a sense of calm and order, contributing to a restful sleep environment. Remove unnecessary items from your bedroom, keeping only the essentials. Consider organizing storage solutions to maintain an uncluttered and serene atmosphere.

6. Temperature Control:

Temperature can significantly impact sleep quality. Aim to keep your bedroom cool, as a slightly lower temperature is generally more conducive to sleep. Experiment with bedding layers that allow you to adjust to your preferred level of warmth. Additionally, consider using a fan or adjusting your thermostat to create an optimal sleep climate.

7. White Noise or Soundscapes:

External noises can disrupt sleep and affect its overall quality. Consider incorporating white noise machines or nature soundscapes to mask disruptive sounds. Alternatively, earplugs may be useful in minimizing disturbances if noise is unavoidable.

8. Establishing a Sleep Routine:

Creating a restful sleep environment goes hand in hand with establishing a consistent sleep routine. Develop pre-sleep rituals such as dimming the lights, engaging in relaxing activities like reading or gentle stretching, and avoiding stimulating screens at least an hour before bedtime. These practices signal to your body that it's time to wind down and prepare for sleep.

9. Personalized Touches:

Incorporate personalized touches that resonate with a sense of calm and comfort. This could include soft, cozy blankets, soothing artwork, or scents like lavender, known for its relaxation-inducing properties. Personalizing your sleep space makes it uniquely yours and enhances the overall sense of tranquility.

10. Evaluating and Adjusting:

Creating a restful sleep environment is an ongoing process. Periodically evaluate your sleep space and make adjustments based on your evolving needs. Consider factors such as changes in seasons, lifestyle, or personal preferences to ensure your bedroom remains a sanctuary for restorative sleep.

Conclusion:

Crafting a restful sleep environment is a foundational step towards improving the quality of your sleep and, consequently, your overall well-being. By attending to the physical and sensory aspects of your bedroom, you create a haven for relaxation and rejuvenation. As we navigate the subsequent chapters, we will explore additional strategies, sleep hygiene practices, and lifestyle adjustments that complement the creation of an optimal sleep environment, setting the stage for restful nights and revitalized days. Remember, the investment you make in your sleep environment pays dividends in the form of improved health, mood, and cognitive function.

Chapter 6: Building a Supportive Community

The Importance of Social Support in Achieving Wellness Goals

In the pursuit of wellness goals, the role of social support cannot be overstated. Whether aiming for weight loss, adopting healthier habits, or enhancing overall well-being, the connections we cultivate with others significantly influence our journey. This chapter explores the multifaceted importance of social support, from motivation and accountability to emotional well-being, providing insights into how building a supportive network can be a game-changer in achieving and sustaining wellness objectives.

1. Motivation and Encouragement:

Embarking on a journey towards wellness often requires a considerable amount of motivation. Having a supportive network provides a source of inspiration and encouragement. Friends, family, or even online communities can offer words of motivation, share success stories, and provide a positive environment that fuels your determination. Knowing that others believe in your capabilities can be a powerful force in overcoming challenges and staying committed to your goals.

2. Accountability and Consistency:

One of the key benefits of social support is the element of accountability. When you share your wellness goals with others, there is a sense of responsibility to stay consistent and true to your objectives. Whether it's a workout buddy waiting at the gym, a friend joining you in healthier meal choices, or a group tracking progress together, the accountability factor reinforces the commitment to your wellness journey.

3. Emotional Well-Being and Stress Reduction:

The connection between social support and emotional well-being is profound. Wellness is not solely about physical health; it encompasses mental and emotional aspects as well. Having a supportive network provides an outlet for sharing thoughts and feelings, reducing stress, and fostering a sense of belonging. During challenging times, knowing that you have a circle of individuals who understand and empathize can be a crucial buffer against the emotional toll of wellness journeys.

4. Shared Learning and Resources:

Building a network of individuals with similar wellness goals opens doors to shared learning and resource-sharing. Whether it's discovering new workout routines, swapping healthy recipes, or discussing effective stress management techniques, the collective knowledge of a supportive community can enhance your own understanding and implementation of wellness strategies.

5. Overcoming Challenges Together:

Wellness journeys are not linear, and challenges are an inevitable part of the process. Having a supportive network allows you to navigate obstacles collectively. Shared experiences of setbacks and triumphs create a sense of camaraderie, providing valuable insights and strategies for overcoming challenges. This shared resilience reinforces the idea that setbacks are temporary, and success is a collective endeavor.

6. Social Influence on Habits and Lifestyle:

The people we surround ourselves with significantly impact our habits and lifestyle choices. If those within our social circle prioritize wellness, it becomes a norm rather than an exception. Social influence can motivate individuals to adopt healthier habits, such as regular exercise, mindful eating, and stress reduction practices. Conversely, being in an environment that fosters unhealthy behaviors can hinder wellness goals.

7. Building Supportive Environments:

Intentionally cultivating a supportive environment involves both seeking out like-minded individuals and fostering a culture of encouragement. Whether it's creating wellness challenges at the workplace, joining community fitness classes, or participating in online forums, the act of building supportive environments contributes to the sustained success of wellness goals.

8. Celebrating Achievements Together:

Success is more meaningful when shared. Celebrating achievements, no matter how small, with a supportive network enhances the joy of accomplishment. Whether it's reaching a weight loss milestone, completing a fitness challenge, or adopting a new healthy habit, the collective celebration reinforces a positive mindset and motivates further progress.

Conclusion:

In the tapestry of wellness, social support is a thread that weaves connections, reinforces commitment, and enriches the overall experience. Recognizing the importance of building a supportive network and actively seeking out connections that align with your wellness goals is a transformative step. As we delve into the subsequent chapters, practical strategies for cultivating social support, effective communication, and overcoming potential barriers will be explored. Remember, the journey towards wellness is not a solitary endeavor but a shared expedition towards a healthier, happier life.

Connecting with Like-Minded Individuals: Building a Supportive Community for Your Wellness Journey

In the pursuit of health and well-being, the power of community cannot be overstated. Connecting with like-minded individuals provides a valuable support system that can significantly enhance your wellness journey. This chapter explores the importance of social connections, strategies for building a supportive community, and the transformative impact of shared experiences on your path to a healthier lifestyle.

1. The Impact of Social Connections on Well-being:

Human beings are inherently social creatures, and our connections with others play a profound role in shaping our well-being. Research consistently highlights the positive impact of social interactions on mental and physical health. When it comes to embarking on a wellness journey, having a supportive network can provide encouragement, motivation, and a sense of belonging, making the path to health more enjoyable and sustainable.

2. The Supportive Power of Like-Minded Individuals:

Like-minded individuals share similar goals, values, and aspirations. When you connect with others who are on a similar wellness journey, you create a supportive environment where challenges are understood, victories are celebrated, and the collective energy propels everyone forward. This shared experience fosters a sense of camaraderie, reducing feelings of isolation and enhancing your overall resilience.

3. Strategies for Building a Supportive Community:

- Join Online Communities: The digital age has facilitated the creation of online communities centered around health and wellness. Platforms like social media groups, forums, and wellness apps offer spaces to connect with individuals who share your goals. Engaging in discussions, sharing experiences, and seeking advice from these online communities can be both informative and uplifting.

- Attend Fitness Classes or Group Activities: Participating in fitness classes, group workouts, or wellness events not only enhances physical health but also provides opportunities to connect with like-minded individuals. The shared experience of pushing towards common fitness goals creates a sense of unity and shared achievement.

- Local Meetups and Support Groups: Look for local meetups or support groups focused on health and wellness. Whether it's a walking group, cooking class, or a mindfulness workshop, these gatherings offer a chance to connect with people who prioritize well-being.

- Create Your Own Support Network: If you can't find an existing community that aligns with your goals, consider creating your own. Invite friends, family, or colleagues to join you in your wellness journey. Having a personal support network can be incredibly motivating and strengthens your commitment to positive lifestyle changes.

4. THE TRANSFORMATIVE Impact of Shared Experiences:

Sharing your wellness journey with others not only provides accountability but also amplifies the joy of successes and lessens the weight of challenges. Whether it's conquering a fitness milestone, trying a new recipe, or overcoming a setback, having like-minded individuals to share these experiences makes the journey more meaningful and enjoyable.

5. Emotional Support and Encouragement:

Wellness is not just about physical health; it encompasses emotional well-being too. Like-minded individuals can offer emotional support, understanding the highs and lows of the journey. Encouraging words, shared tips, and empathetic conversations create a positive atmosphere that fuels your determination and resilience.

6. Overcoming Challenges Together:

Every wellness journey comes with its set of challenges. Whether it's breaking through a fitness plateau, overcoming cravings, or navigating emotional hurdles, facing these challenges alongside supportive individuals can make the difference between persistence and giving up. The collective strength of a community can help you push past obstacles and stay focused on your goals.

Conclusion:

Connecting with like-minded individuals is a transformative aspect of your wellness journey. As you build a supportive community, you not only enhance your chances of success but also create a network that enriches your life beyond physical health. The subsequent chapters will explore additional strategies for maintaining and deepening these connections, ensuring that your wellness community becomes a lasting source of inspiration, motivation, and joy. Remember, you are not alone on this journey, and the bonds you form with others can be a powerful catalyst for positive change in your life.

Overcoming Challenges Together: The Power of Support in Weight Loss

Embarking on a weight loss journey can be a transformative yet challenging experience. The road to sustainable change is often dotted with obstacles that can test your resolve and motivation. In this chapter, we explore the profound impact of social support, strategies for building a supportive community, and the strength that comes from facing challenges together.

1. The Impact of Social Support:

Weight loss is not a solitary endeavor; the influence of social connections can be a driving force behind success. Whether it's friends, family, or like-minded individuals sharing a similar journey, having a support system in place provides encouragement, accountability, and a shared sense of purpose. Studies consistently show that individuals with strong social support are more likely to achieve and maintain their weight loss goals.

2. Building Your Support Network:

Creating a support network involves intentional efforts to surround yourself with individuals who uplift and encourage your journey. This network can include:

- Friends and Family: Share your goals with those close to you. Their understanding, encouragement, and willingness to engage in healthy activities can be a powerful motivator.

- Online Communities: Joining online forums, social media groups, or weight loss communities allows you to connect with a broader network of individuals who share similar goals. The exchange of experiences, tips, and encouragement in these spaces can be invaluable.

- Accountability Partners: Forming partnerships with friends or family members who are also on a health and wellness journey creates a sense of shared commitment. Regular check-ins, joint workouts, or cooking healthy meals together can strengthen the bond and make the journey more enjoyable.

3. The Role of Emotional Support:

Weight loss is not just a physical transformation; it involves navigating emotional challenges as well. Having emotional support can help you cope with stress, setbacks, and the emotional aspects of the journey. Whether it's a trusted friend, family member, or professional counselor, having someone to talk to can provide valuable perspective and encouragement.

4. Joint Goal Setting and Celebration:

Setting shared goals with your support network creates a sense of camaraderie and collective achievement. Celebrate milestones together, whether it's reaching a certain weight, completing a fitness challenge, or adopting a new healthy habit. Joint celebrations reinforce the idea that success is a shared experience, fostering motivation for the journey ahead.

5. Effective Communication:

Open and honest communication is crucial within your support network. Clearly express your needs, goals, and challenges, and be receptive to feedback and suggestions. Establishing a foundation of understanding and empathy ensures that your support system can provide assistance tailored to your individual journey.

6. Overcoming Obstacles as a Team:

Challenges are inevitable on the path to weight loss, and facing them together can make overcoming obstacles more manageable. Whether it's navigating social events, dealing with emotional triggers, or adapting to lifestyle changes, having a supportive community provides varied perspectives, strategies, and encouragement to help you overcome hurdles.

7. Group Activities and Fitness Classes:

Engaging in group activities or fitness classes not only contributes to physical well-being but also fosters a sense of community. Whether it's a group workout, a dance class, or a hiking club, participating in activities together creates shared experiences and strengthens the bonds within your support network.

8. Empathy and Non-Judgmental Support:

Creating a supportive environment involves cultivating empathy and non-judgmental support. Everyone's journey is unique, and individuals may face different challenges. Offering understanding and encouragement without judgment creates a safe space where everyone feels valued and supported.

Conclusion:

The journey to weight loss is not meant to be traveled alone. The power of overcoming challenges together lies in the shared experiences, encouragement, and collective strength that a support network provides. As you navigate the chapters ahead, consider how you can build and leverage your support system to enhance your journey. Remember, the challenges you face are not obstacles but opportunities for growth, and facing them together with a supportive community makes the path more rewarding and sustainable.

Chapter 7: Tracking Progress and Staying Motivated

Setting Milestones and Celebrating Achievements: A Blueprint for Success

In the pursuit of any significant goal, including weight loss, setting milestones and celebrating achievements serves as a powerful motivational tool. This chapter delves into the importance of establishing meaningful milestones, the role they play in maintaining momentum, and how celebrating achievements contributes to a positive and sustainable journey.

1. The Significance of Milestones:

Milestones are like guideposts on the path to success, providing direction and marking progress. They break down the overarching goal into manageable and measurable components, making the journey more achievable and less overwhelming. Instead of focusing solely on the ultimate destination, setting milestones encourages individuals to celebrate the small victories along the way.

2. Creating SMART Milestones:

Just as with goal-setting, milestones benefit from the SMART criteria: Specific, Measurable, Achievable, Relevant, and Time-bound. Specific milestones clearly define what you want to achieve, measurable milestones allow for progress tracking, achievable milestones are realistic, relevant milestones align with your overall goals, and time-bound milestones provide a timeframe for completion. Applying these criteria ensures that your milestones are well-defined and conducive to success.

3. Short-Term vs. Long-Term Milestones:

Breaking down your weight loss journey into short-term and long-term milestones is essential for maintaining focus and motivation. Short-term milestones may include achieving a certain number of steps per day, consistently following a workout routine, or incorporating more vegetables into your meals. Long-term milestones encompass larger goals like reaching a specific weight, completing a fitness challenge, or achieving a significant health improvement. Both types of milestones contribute to a sense of accomplishment and progress.

4. The Psychological Impact:

Milestones have a profound psychological impact on individuals. Achieving a milestone triggers a sense of accomplishment, boosting confidence, and reinforcing the belief that progress is possible. This positive reinforcement contributes to a resilient mindset, fostering the motivation needed to overcome challenges and setbacks.

5. Celebrating Achievements:

Celebrating achievements is not merely a self-indulgent act; it is a crucial aspect of the journey. Recognizing and celebrating milestones, whether big or small, creates a positive feedback loop that enhances motivation and commitment. Celebration doesn't have to be extravagant; it can be as simple as acknowledging your progress, treating yourself to a non-food-related reward, or sharing your achievements with a supportive community.

6. CULTIVATING A POSITIVE Relationship with Progress:

Setting milestones and celebrating achievements contribute to cultivating a positive relationship with progress. It shifts the focus from what hasn't been achieved to what has, creating an optimistic outlook that is essential for long-term success. Rather than fixating on the distance still to be covered, individuals can appreciate how far they've come, reinforcing a sense of self-efficacy and determination.

7. Adapting Milestones Along the Way:

Flexibility in milestone-setting is crucial to adapt to the evolving nature of the journey. As circumstances change, goals may need to be adjusted. Being open to reassessing and modifying milestones ensures that they remain relevant and achievable, preventing frustration in the face of unforeseen challenges.

8. Building a Supportive Community:

Sharing your milestones and celebrating achievements with a supportive community enhances the joy of success. Whether it's friends, family, or fellow individuals on a similar journey, a community provides encouragement, accountability, and shared victories. Celebrating achievements together strengthens the sense of connection and mutual support.

Conclusion:

Setting milestones and celebrating achievements is not a mere formality; it is a dynamic and essential component of a successful weight loss journey. By breaking down the overarching goal into manageable steps, individuals create a roadmap that not only guides them towards success but also enhances their motivation and resilience. The subsequent chapters will explore practical strategies for setting meaningful milestones, overcoming common challenges, and cultivating a positive mindset that propels you towards continued achievements. Remember, every step forward is a victory, and every milestone reached is a cause for celebration on the transformative path to lasting well-being.

Adjusting Strategies as Needed: Navigating the Dynamic Path of Weight Management

In the journey of weight management, adaptability is a key virtue. This chapter explores the importance of adjusting strategies as needed, acknowledging the dynamic nature of individual circumstances, evolving goals, and the ever-changing landscape of life. From recognizing signs that warrant adjustment to practical approaches for refining your approach, this discussion aims to empower you with the flexibility to navigate your unique path successfully.

1. Recognizing Signs for Adjustment:

Weight management is not a linear process, and recognizing signs that indicate the need for adjustment is crucial for long-term success. Common indicators may include:

- Plateaus: If weight loss stalls despite consistent efforts, it may be time to reassess your approach.

- Life Changes: Significant life events, such as job changes, family dynamics, or health issues, can impact your routine and require adjustments to your strategies.

- Mental and Emotional Well-being: Changes in stress levels, emotional well-being, or mental health may influence eating habits and exercise patterns, necessitating a tailored approach.

- Physical Health: Modifications may be needed if there are changes in your physical health, such as injuries, illnesses, or alterations in metabolism.

2. The Art of Self-Reflection:

Regular self-reflection is a powerful tool for assessing the effectiveness of your current strategies. Consider journaling about your experiences, emotions, and challenges related to weight management. This practice helps you gain insights into patterns, triggers, and areas that may require adjustment. Self-reflection also fosters a mindful awareness of your journey, promoting a positive and proactive mindset.

3. Adapting Nutritional Strategies:

Dietary adjustments are often necessary as your body and goals evolve. This may involve:

- Caloric Intake: Recalculate your daily caloric needs based on changes in weight, activity level, and metabolism.

- Macronutrient Balance: Adjust the proportions of carbohydrates, proteins, and fats to meet your current needs and goals.

- Meal Timing: Experiment with meal timing to optimize energy levels and support your lifestyle. This could involve adjusting the frequency and timing of meals and snacks.

4. Fine-Tuning Exercise Routines:

Physical activity is a cornerstone of weight management, but as circumstances change, so too should your exercise routine. Consider:

- Intensity and Duration: Modify the intensity and duration of workouts to align with your fitness level, preventing burnout or excessive strain.

- Variety: Introduce variety into your workouts to prevent monotony and challenge your body in new ways. This could include trying different types of exercise or incorporating cross-training.

- Consistency: Ensure consistency in your exercise routine, even if adjustments are needed. Regular physical activity contributes not only to weight management but also to overall health and well-being.

5. Addressing Emotional and Mental Well-being:

Emotional and mental well-being are integral components of successful weight management. Adjusting strategies in this realm involves:

- Stress Management: Implement stress-reducing practices such as mindfulness, meditation, or activities that bring joy.

- Seeking Support: If emotional or mental health challenges arise, consider seeking support from professionals such as therapists, counselors, or support groups.

- Mindful Eating Practices: Reconnect with mindful eating habits, paying attention to hunger and fullness cues, and addressing emotional triggers.

6. Setting Realistic and Adjusted Goals:

As you adapt your strategies, revisiting and adjusting your goals is equally important. Setting realistic and achievable goals based on your current circumstances ensures that you maintain motivation and a positive outlook. Celebrate milestones, no matter how small, and use them as stepping stones for continued progress.

7. Seeking Professional Guidance:

When in doubt, seeking guidance from health professionals such as dietitians, fitness trainers, or mental health experts can provide tailored advice based on your individual needs. These professionals can offer support, monitor progress, and guide adjustments that align with your goals and overall well-being.

Conclusion:

Adjusting strategies as needed is not a sign of failure but a testament to your adaptability and commitment to long-term well-being. Embrace the dynamic nature of your weight management journey, viewing adjustments as opportunities for growth and refinement. The subsequent chapters will delve into specific challenges and offer practical guidance on adapting strategies in various scenarios. Remember, the ability to adjust, learn, and persevere is the hallmark of a successful weight management journey that evolves with you, ensuring sustained success and well-being.

Cultivating Long-Term Motivation

In the realm of weight management and wellness, motivation is the fuel that propels individuals on their journey. Yet, the challenge lies not only in finding the initial spark but in cultivating a sustainable flame that withstands the test of time. This chapter explores the dynamics of long-term motivation, offering insights into understanding, fostering, and maintaining the drive to pursue health and well-being consistently.

1. Understanding Motivation:

Motivation is a complex interplay of internal and external factors that drive individuals to initiate and sustain actions towards their goals. It's crucial to recognize that motivation is not a constant state; it fluctuates based on circumstances, emotions, and experiences. Understanding the ebb and flow of motivation is the first step in cultivating a long-term commitment to your health journey.

2. Setting Intrinsic Goals:

While external goals, such as achieving a specific weight or fitting into a certain dress size, can be initial motivators, cultivating long-term motivation often requires a shift towards intrinsic goals. Intrinsic motivation arises from personal satisfaction, a sense of accomplishment, and the inherent enjoyment of the process. Focus on goals that align with your values, promote well-being, and contribute to a healthier and happier lifestyle.

3. Creating a Vision and Why:

Establishing a clear vision of what success looks like for you is instrumental in sustaining motivation. Visualize the benefits of your health journey, envision the positive changes in your life, and articulate your "why"—the deep-seated reasons behind your commitment to wellness. Whether it's improved energy, enhanced confidence, or better overall health, a compelling vision and strong "why" serve as powerful motivators during challenging times.

4. Breaking Down Goals into Manageable Steps:

Long-term motivation thrives when goals are broken down into smaller, manageable steps. Instead of fixating on a distant endpoint, focus on achievable milestones that contribute to your larger vision. Celebrate these victories, reinforcing the belief that progress is being made and that the journey is both attainable and rewarding.

5. Embracing Flexibility and Adaptability:

Rigidity can be the nemesis of long-term motivation. Life is dynamic, filled with unexpected challenges and changes. Embrace flexibility in your approach, allowing for adjustments to your goals and strategies as needed. A resilient mindset that adapts to circumstances fosters a sustainable motivation that withstands the inevitable twists and turns of life.

6. Building a Supportive Environment:

Surrounding yourself with a supportive environment is pivotal for maintaining motivation. Share your goals with friends, family, or like-minded individuals who can provide encouragement, understanding, and accountability. A supportive community reinforces your commitment, making the journey more enjoyable and less isolating.

7. Incorporating Enjoyable Activities:

Incorporating activities you enjoy into your health journey adds an element of pleasure and satisfaction, contributing to sustained motivation. Whether it's trying new recipes, engaging in enjoyable workouts, or participating in activities that bring you joy, infusing pleasure into the process enhances long-term commitment.

8. Tracking Progress and Reflecting:

Regularly tracking your progress and reflecting on your journey can be a source of motivation. Recognize the positive changes, no matter how small, and acknowledge the efforts invested. Reflecting on challenges allows for learning and growth, transforming obstacles into stepping stones towards your goals.

9. Reinforcing Positive Habits:

As you progress, focus on reinforcing positive habits. Habits, once ingrained, become automatic and contribute significantly to long-term success. Identify the habits that align with your health goals and consistently practice and reinforce them to build a foundation for lasting well-being.

10. Seeking Professional Guidance:

Sometimes, sustaining motivation requires external support. Seeking guidance from health professionals, such as nutritionists, personal trainers, or therapists, can provide personalized strategies, expertise, and encouragement tailored to your unique journey.

Conclusion:

Cultivating long-term motivation is an ongoing process that evolves with your health journey. By understanding the dynamics of motivation, setting intrinsic goals, creating a compelling vision, and embracing flexibility, individuals can foster a sustained commitment to their well-being. The subsequent chapters will delve into practical strategies for overcoming common obstacles, staying motivated during plateaus, and navigating the complexities of a changing lifestyle. Remember, motivation is not a finite resource; it's a renewable energy that can be nurtured and replenished through intentional actions and a resilient mindset.

8. Conclusion

As we conclude our journey together, "Trimming Triumph" empowers you with the knowledge and tools needed to achieve sustainable weight loss. Remember, it's not just about shedding pounds; it's about embracing a healthier, happier lifestyle. Your triumph is not only in reaching your goal but in maintaining it for the long run. Here's to your success, well-being, and the vibrant life you deserve!

"Success in any endeavor begins with the unwavering belief that your journey is worth the effort.

Embrace each step with determination, knowing that every challenge is an opportunity to prove your resilience. The path to greatness is not without obstacles, but it is those who persist with passion and purpose who leave an indelible mark on the world."
- Unknown

Leading book about Hollistic approach to weight loss strategy.

ISBN 979-8-224-21904-9

Aline Ste-Marie

Les fleurs intérieures

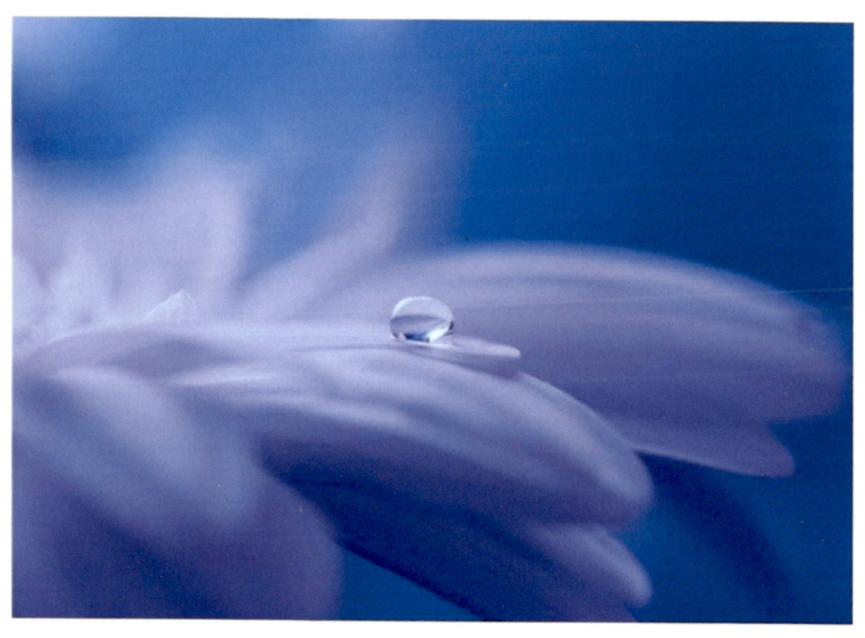

11 nouvelles inspirantes